Weight Training Exercise Made Easy for Beginners

Physical Benefits of Weight Training

By

Paxton Quade

Table of Contents

CHAPTER 1

Introduction

Weight training, also known as strength training or resistance training, is a form of physical exercise that involves lifting weights or using resistance to build and develop muscle strength, endurance, and overall fitness. It has been a cornerstone of fitness and athletic training for centuries and continues to gain popularity for its numerous physical and mental health benefits. we'll delve into the compelling reasons why weight training is a valuable pursuit, particularly for beginners looking to improve their physical well-being.

1.1 Physical Benefits of Weight Training

1. **Muscle Strength and Definition**: One of the primary motivations for individuals to engage in weight training is the desire to build and sculpt lean muscle. Weight training allows you to target specific muscle groups, leading to improved muscle definition and tone. As a beginner, you'll experience noticeable changes in your body composition, which can boost self-confidence and body image.

2. **Increased Metabolism**: Muscle tissue burns more calories at rest than fat tissue. By increasing your lean muscle mass through weight training, you'll elevate your resting

metabolic rate. This means that you'll burn more calories even when you're not working out, making weight management and fat loss more achievable.

3. **Bone Health**: Weight training has a significant positive impact on bone density. As you subject your bones to resistance, they become stronger and more resilient. This is especially important for women and older adults, as it can help prevent or mitigate conditions like osteoporosis.

4. **Improved Posture and Joint Health**: Properly structured weight training programs emphasize functional movements that strengthen the muscles responsible for maintaining good posture and

joint stability. This not only helps prevent injuries but can also alleviate existing joint discomfort.

5. **Enhanced Cardiovascular Health**: While weight training is not primarily a cardiovascular exercise, it can still benefit your heart health. Short rest intervals between sets and high-intensity training can elevate your heart rate, improving cardiovascular fitness.

6. **Injury Prevention**: A well-rounded weight training program incorporates exercises that strengthen both large and small muscle groups. This balanced approach can reduce the risk of injuries by

addressing muscle imbalances and promoting joint stability.

1.2 Mental and Emotional Benefits of Weight Training

1. **Stress Reduction**: Engaging in weight training has been shown to reduce stress and anxiety levels. The physical exertion and the release of endorphins during workouts can have a calming and mood-boosting effect.

2. **Increased Confidence**: As you see progress in your strength and physique, your self-esteem and confidence are likely to soar. Achieving fitness goals

through weight training can be a highly rewarding experience.

3. **Enhanced Mental Focus**: Weight training demands concentration and mental presence, as proper form and technique are essential for safety and effectiveness. This can improve your ability to focus in other areas of your life as well.

4. **Empowerment**: Weight training empowers you to take control of your physical health and fitness. The feeling of becoming stronger and more capable can spill over into other aspects of your life, instilling a sense of empowerment and resilience.

1.3 Accessibility and Versatility

Another compelling reason to consider weight training is its accessibility and versatility. You don't need an expensive gym membership or a vast array of equipment to get started. Basic equipment such as dumbbells, barbells, and resistance bands can provide an effective workout. Moreover, weight training routines can be adapted to suit your goals, whether you're aiming for muscle growth, improved endurance, or fat loss.

weight training is a dynamic and multifaceted exercise modality that offers a wide range of physical, mental, and emotional benefits. For beginners, it serves as an excellent introduction to the world of fitness, offering the opportunity to build a strong foundation for future health and wellness.

CHAPTER 2

Getting Started with Weight Training

Embarking on a weight training journey is an exciting and empowering endeavor. To make the most of your experience and ensure safety, it's essential to lay a solid foundation. This section will guide you through the initial steps of your weight training journey, covering the importance of setting clear goals, choosing the right equipment, and prioritizing safety precautions.

2.1 Setting Clear Goals

Before you dive into weight training, it's crucial to set clear and achievable goals. Your goals act as a roadmap, keeping you motivated and on track throughout your fitness journey. Here are some key considerations when setting your weight training goals:

1. **Specificity**: Define your objectives in precise terms. Instead of a vague goal like "get in shape," specify what "getting in shape" means to you. For instance, it could be "increase muscle mass," "improve strength," or "lose body fat."

2. **Measurability**: Ensure that your goals are measurable. You should be able to track your progress over time. This might

involve recording the weight you lift, the number of repetitions you can perform, or changes in your body measurements.

3. **Realistic and Attainable**: While it's great to aim high, your goals should also be realistic and attainable. Setting unattainable goals can lead to frustration and discouragement. Base your goals on your current fitness level and the time you can realistically commit to training.

4. **Time-Bound**: Set a timeframe for achieving your goals. This could be weeks, months, or even years. A timeline helps create a sense of urgency and allows you to measure your progress.

5. **Long-Term and Short-Term Goals**: Consider both long-term and short-term goals. Long-term goals might involve substantial changes, while short-term goals can help you stay motivated and focused along the way.

6. **Adaptability**: Be open to adjusting your goals as your fitness journey unfolds. As you gain experience, you may find that your priorities evolve. Flexibility in your goals allows you to adapt to changing circumstances.

Once you've set your goals, write them down and keep them visible. This visual reminder can help keep you accountable and motivated as you progress in your weight training program.

2.2 Choosing the Right Equipment

Selecting the appropriate equipment for your weight training regimen is crucial to your success. While there are various options available, you don't need an elaborate setup to get started. Here's how to choose the right equipment:

1. **Free Weights vs. Machines**: Beginners often wonder whether to start with free weights (dumbbells and barbells) or weight machines. Free weights offer a more comprehensive and functional workout, engaging stabilizer muscles, while machines provide more stability. As a beginner, it's beneficial to incorporate both into your routine.

2. **Start with the Basics**: As a novice, focus on fundamental equipment. A set of dumbbells, a barbell with weight plates, a bench, and resistance bands are excellent choices. These items allow you to perform a wide range of exercises.

3. **Consider Your Space**: Depending on your available space, you may opt for home equipment or a gym membership. If you're working out at home, ensure you have enough space to move comfortably and store your equipment.

4. **Quality Matters**: Invest in quality equipment that's safe and durable. It's better to have a few high-quality items than a

vast collection of subpar equipment.

5. **Consult a Professional**: If you're uncertain about your equipment choices, consider seeking advice from a fitness professional or personal trainer. They can help you select the best gear based on your goals and budget.

2.3 Safety Precautions

Safety is paramount in weight training, especially for beginners. Here are essential safety precautions to keep in mind:

1. **Proper Warm-Up**: Always begin your workout with a proper warm-up. This can include light cardio, dynamic

stretching, and mobility exercises. A warm-up prepares your body for the demands of weight training and reduces the risk of injury.

2. **Learn Proper Form**: Correct form is crucial to prevent injuries and ensure the effectiveness of your exercises. Prioritize learning the proper technique for each exercise. Consider working with a qualified trainer to get guidance.

3. **Start with Manageable Weights**: Begin with weights that you can lift comfortably with good form. Don't attempt to lift heavy weights before you've mastered the basics.

4. **Use Spotters**: When lifting heavy weights, especially during exercises like bench press and squats, have a spotter present to assist you in case you need help.

5. **Progress Gradually**: Avoid the temptation to increase weight rapidly. Gradual progression is safer and more sustainable. Aim for small increments in weight or repetitions over time.

6. **Stay Hydrated and Rest**: Proper hydration is essential for optimal performance and recovery. Ensure you get adequate rest between sets and between workouts to allow your muscles to recover.

7. **Listen to Your Body**: Pay attention to any pain or discomfort. If you experience pain beyond normal muscle soreness, stop the exercise immediately and seek guidance if needed.

8. **Consult a Healthcare Professional**: If you have any underlying health conditions or concerns, consult with a healthcare professional before starting a weight training program.

Getting started with weight training is an exciting endeavor, but it's essential to begin with a clear understanding of your goals, the right equipment, and a strong focus on safety. These initial steps will set you on a path to a successful and injury-free weight training journey.

CHAPTER 3

Understanding the Basics

Before diving into weight training, it's important to grasp the fundamental concepts that underpin effective and safe workouts. This section provides an overview of the basics, covering the anatomy and muscle groups involved, the different types of weight training exercises, and the critical components of repetitions, sets, and rest periods.

3.1 Anatomy and Muscle Groups

Understanding the anatomy and the major muscle groups in the human body is crucial for effective weight training. The knowledge of muscle groups helps you target specific areas and create a balanced workout routine. Here are some key muscle groups:

1. **Chest Muscles (Pectorals)**: These muscles are responsible for movements like bench presses and push-ups.

2. **Back Muscles (Latissimus Dorsi and Trapezius)**: The back muscles are engaged in exercises like rows and pull-ups, aiding in posture and upper body strength.

3. **Shoulder Muscles (Deltoids)**: The deltoid muscles are involved in overhead presses and lateral raises.

4. **Arm Muscles (Biceps and Triceps)**: Bicep curls and tricep extensions target these muscles and contribute to arm strength.

5. **Leg Muscles (Quadriceps, Hamstrings, Calves)**: Squats and lunges work the quadriceps and hamstrings, while calf raises target the calf muscles.

6. **Core Muscles (Abdominals and Lower Back)**: Core strength is essential for stability and balance. Exercises like planks and crunches strengthen the core.

7. **Gluteal Muscles (Glutes)**: Squats and deadlifts engage the

glutes, contributing to overall lower body strength.

Understanding the function and location of these muscle groups will help you tailor your workouts to your fitness goals and ensure a well-rounded training routine. It's important to note that many weight training exercises engage multiple muscle groups simultaneously, promoting functional strength and overall fitness.

3.2 Types of Weight Training Exercises

Weight training encompasses a wide variety of exercises, each with its own benefits and applications. Here are some common types of weight training exercises:

1. **Compound Exercises**: These exercises engage multiple muscle groups simultaneously. Examples include squats, deadlifts, bench presses, and rows. Compound exercises are highly effective for building overall strength and muscle mass.

2. **Isolation Exercises**: Isolation exercises target specific muscle groups. Examples include bicep curls, tricep extensions, and leg extensions. These exercises are useful for focusing on a particular muscle group and addressing muscle imbalances.

3. **Bodyweight Exercises**: While not using traditional weights, bodyweight exercises like push-ups, pull-ups, and planks are effective for building

strength and improving endurance. They are particularly beneficial for beginners and can be performed anywhere.

4. **Functional Training**: Functional exercises replicate movements used in daily life or sports. These exercises enhance overall coordination and agility. Examples include medicine ball throws and cable wood chops.

5. **Plyometrics**: Plyometric exercises involve explosive movements, often with jumping or hopping. They improve power and athleticism. Plyometric exercises include box jumps, squat jumps, and burpees.

6. **Machine-Based Exercises**:
   Weight machines at the gym
   can be beneficial for beginners
   as they provide stability and
   guidance for proper form.
   Machines target specific muscle
   groups and are often easy to
   use.

The choice of exercises should align with your goals and your current fitness level. For beginners, it's advisable to start with a mix of compound and isolation exercises to build a solid foundation.

3.3 Reps, Sets, and Rest Periods

Repetitions (reps), sets, and rest periods are key components of a weight training workout:

1. **Repetitions (Reps)**:
   Repetitions refer to the number
   of times you perform a specific
   exercise. The ideal number of
   reps varies depending on your
   goals. Higher reps (e.g., 12-15)
   with lower weight emphasize
   muscle endurance, while lower
   reps (e.g., 6-8) with heavier
   weights focus on muscle
   strength.

2. **Sets**: A set is a group of
   repetitions performed
   consecutively. Beginners
   typically start with 2-4 sets per
   exercise. The number of sets
   can be adjusted to match your
   fitness level and goals.

3. **Rest Periods**: Rest periods
   between sets are important.
   Shorter rest periods (e.g., 30-60
   seconds) promote muscular

endurance and calorie burn, while longer rest periods (e.g., 2-3 minutes) are essential for muscle recovery and strength building.

Understanding these fundamentals helps you structure your workouts effectively. For strength and muscle building, consider a typical approach of 3-4 sets of 8-12 reps with 1-2 minutes of rest between sets. As your fitness level advances, you can adjust these variables to suit your goals and training capacity.

a solid understanding of anatomy, muscle groups, types of weight training exercises, and the components of reps, sets, and rest periods is essential for creating a well-rounded and effective weight training program.

CHAPTER 4

Essential Weight Training Exercises

A well-rounded weight training program includes a selection of essential exercises that target various muscle groups and promote overall strength and fitness. These exercises form the foundation of many workout routines, and mastering them is key to achieving your fitness goals.

4.1 Squats

Squats are often referred to as the "king of exercises" due to their effectiveness in working multiple muscle groups and improving overall strength. They primarily target the quadriceps, hamstrings, glutes, lower back, and core. Here's how to perform squats:

1. **Starting Position**: Stand with your feet shoulder-width apart. Keep your chest up, shoulders back, and your head in a neutral position.

2. **Movement**: Begin by pushing your hips back and bending your knees. Lower your body as if you were sitting back into a chair. Keep your knees aligned with your feet and your back straight.

3. **Depth**: Go as low as your flexibility and strength allow, ideally until your thighs are parallel to the ground or lower.

Maintain a neutral spine throughout the movement.

4. **Ascent**: Push through your heels to stand back up, returning to the starting position.

Squats build lower body strength, improve core stability, and contribute to better posture and balance. They can be performed with a barbell, dumbbells, or body weight.

4.2 Deadlifts

Deadlifts are another essential compound exercise that primarily targets the glutes, hamstrings, lower back, and the entire posterior chain. Proper form is crucial to prevent injury. Here's how to perform the conventional deadlift:

1. **Starting Position**: Stand with your feet hip-width apart, toes under the barbell. Bend at your hips and knees to lower yourself, keeping your back straight and your chest up. Grip the barbell with both hands, hands just outside your knees.

2. **Lift**: With your core engaged and back straight, lift the bar by extending your hips and knees simultaneously. Keep the barbell close to your body as you stand up.

3. **Lockout**: Stand tall with your shoulders back and your hips fully extended. Hold the barbell for a moment before lowering it back to the ground.

Deadlifts are excellent for developing strength and power, particularly in the lower body and the muscles of the back. They can also be performed with variations like the sumo deadlift or trap bar deadlift.

4.3 Bench Press

The *bench press* is a classic upper body exercise that targets the chest, shoulders, and triceps. It's an essential compound movement for building upper body strength and muscle mass. Here's how to perform the bench press:

1. **Starting Position**: Lie on your back on a bench with your feet flat on the ground. Grip the barbell slightly wider than shoulder-width apart, arms fully extended. Your eyes should be directly under the barbell.

2. **Descent**: Lower the bar to your chest in a controlled manner. Keep your elbows at a 45-degree angle to your torso, and ensure your wrists are straight.

3. **Ascent**: Push the barbell back up to the starting position, fully extending your arms.

Bench presses can be performed with a barbell or dumbbells, and they are crucial for building chest strength and size. Proper form is essential to avoid injury and maximize results.

4.4 Rows

Rows are an important upper body exercise that targets the muscles of the back, including the lats and rhomboids, as well as the biceps.

Here's how to perform bent-over barbell rows, a common variation:

1. **Starting Position**: Stand with your feet hip-width apart and hold a barbell in front of your thighs, palms facing you. Bend at your hips to lower your torso until it's nearly parallel to the ground. Keep your back straight, core engaged, and knees slightly bent.

2. **Row**: Pull the barbell toward your lower ribcage, squeezing your shoulder blades together. Keep your elbows close to your body. Hold the position briefly.

3. **Lower**: Extend your arms to return the barbell to the starting position.

Rows are effective for building a strong and well-developed back, which is essential for good posture and overall upper body strength.

4.5 Overhead Press

The *overhead press*, also known as the shoulder press or military press, targets the deltoid muscles of the shoulders and the triceps. It's an excellent exercise for building upper body strength and shoulder stability. Here's how to perform the overhead press:

1. **Starting Position**: Stand with your feet hip-width apart. Grip a barbell or dumbbells with your palms facing forward and the weight at shoulder level.

2. **Press**: Push the weight overhead by extending your arms, but be sure not to lock

your elbows. Keep your core
engaged to support your lower
back.

3. **Lockout**: Fully extend your
   arms overhead, and then lower
   the weight back to shoulder
   level.

The overhead press is effective for
building shoulder strength and
increasing overhead stability, making
it a fundamental upper body exercise.

Incorporating these essential weight
training exercises into your workout
routine will help you build a strong
and balanced physique. Be sure to
start with proper form, and gradually
increase the weight as your strength
and confidence grow.

4.6 Bicep Curls

Bicep curls are isolation exercises that specifically target the biceps, the muscles on the front of your upper arms. These exercises help build arm strength and improve the aesthetics of your biceps. Here's how to perform a basic standing dumbbell bicep curl:

1. **Starting Position**: Stand with your feet shoulder-width apart, holding a dumbbell in each hand with your palms facing forward. Your arms should be fully extended by your sides.

2. **Curl**: While keeping your upper arms stationary and your back straight, bend your elbows to curl the dumbbells towards your shoulders. Squeeze your biceps at the top of the movement.

3. **Lower**: Slowly lower the dumbbells back to the starting position, fully extending your arms.

4.7 Tricep Extensions

Tricep extensions, or tricep press-downs, focus on the triceps, the muscles on the back of your upper arms. Strong triceps are essential for pushing movements and overall arm strength. Here's how to perform tricep press-downs using a cable machine:

1. **Starting Position**: Stand in front of a cable machine with a straight bar attached to the high pulley. Grasp the bar with both hands, palms facing down. Keep your feet hip-width apart.

2. **Extension**: With your elbows close to your body, extend your arms downward to fully straighten them. Your triceps should contract at the bottom of the movement.

3. **Return**: Slowly bring the bar back to the starting position, bending your elbows.

Tricep extensions can also be performed with a rope attachment or a V-bar. They are excellent for developing tricep strength and improving the appearance of the back of your arms.

4.8 Core Strengthening Exercises

Core strengthening exercises are vital for building a stable and resilient midsection. A strong core is not only essential for overall strength but also for maintaining good posture and preventing injuries. Here are some core-strengthening exercises:

1. **Plank**: Start in a push-up position with your weight supported on your forearms and toes. Keep your body in a straight line from head to heels, engaging your core muscles. Hold the position for as long as you can while maintaining proper form.

2. **Russian Twists**: Sit on the floor with your knees bent, lean back slightly, and lift your feet off the ground. Hold a weight or a medicine ball with both hands and twist your torso to one side, then the other. This exercise engages the oblique muscles.

3. **Leg Raises**: Lie on your back with your legs straight. Lift your legs off the ground by flexing your hips and raising your feet toward the ceiling. Lower them back down without letting them touch the ground. This exercise targets the lower abdominal muscles.

4. **Superman**: Lie face down with your arms extended in front of you and your legs straight. Lift your arms, chest, and legs off the ground simultaneously, forming a "flying" position. Hold briefly and lower back down.

5. **Hanging Leg Raise**: Hang from a pull-up bar or a sturdy horizontal surface. Raise your legs while keeping them straight. Lift them as high as

you can, engaging your lower abdominal muscles.

Incorporate these core-strengthening exercises into your weight training routine to improve core stability, balance, and overall functional strength. A strong core is essential for maintaining proper form in other weight training exercises and daily activities.

This essential weight training exercises, including bicep curls, tricep extensions, and core-strengthening exercises, offer a balanced approach to building strength and muscle definition. When combined with the previously discussed fundamental exercises, they form a well-rounded workout routine that can be adapted to meet your fitness goals and preferences.

CHAPTER 5

Creating Your Workout Routine

5.1 Designing a Beginner-Friendly Workout Plan

Designing a workout plan for beginners is about balance, progression, and sustainability. Here are the key steps to create a beginner-friendly workout plan:

Step 1: Set Clear Goals: Start by defining your fitness goals. Whether it's building muscle, losing weight, increasing strength, or improving overall fitness, knowing your objectives will guide your workout plan.

Step 2: Choose the Right Exercises: Incorporate a variety of exercises that target different muscle groups. Include compound exercises like squats, deadlifts, bench presses, rows, and overhead presses, as well as isolation exercises like bicep curls and tricep extensions. Don't forget core-strengthening exercises.

Step 3: Create a Balanced Routine: Balance your workouts by including both upper and lower body exercises, as well as exercises for different muscle groups. Aim for a routine that works the whole body over the course of a week.

Step 4: Plan Your Training Split: Decide how often you'll work out. A typical beginner's split might be three full-body workouts per week, with a rest day between each session. This allows for adequate recovery.

Step 5: Determine Reps and Sets: Begin with 2-4 sets of each exercise with 8-12 repetitions (reps) per set. This range is a good starting point for building both strength and muscle endurance.

Step 6: Focus on Form and Technique: Prioritize learning and maintaining proper form to prevent injury and maximize results. Consider working with a trainer or watching instructional videos to ensure you're doing exercises correctly.

Step 7: Warm-Up and Cool Down: Always warm up with light cardio and dynamic stretching before your workout. Finish with static stretching and a cool-down to aid recovery.

Step 8: Incorporate Rest Days: Rest days are crucial for recovery. Your muscles need time to repair and grow. Don't neglect rest days in your routine.

Step 9: Progression: Over time, gradually increase the weight, repetitions, or intensity of your workouts to promote continuous progress. This leads us to the principle of progressive overload.

5.2 Progressive Overload

Progressive overload is a fundamental concept in weight training. It involves gradually increasing the demands placed on your muscles to encourage growth and improvement. Here's how to implement progressive overload:

1. **Increase Weight**: As you become comfortable with a particular weight, gradually add more resistance. This can be done by using heavier dumbbells, barbells, or weight plates.

2. **Add Reps**: When you can perform the recommended number of repetitions with good form, try to do one or two more reps in each set. This gradually increases the intensity of your workouts.

3. **Adjust Sets**: You can also add an additional set to your exercises, which increases the overall volume of your workout and challenges your muscles further.

4. **Shorten Rest Periods**:
    Reducing rest periods between
    sets can make your workouts
    more intense and encourage
    muscle adaptation.

5. **Vary Exercises**: Incorporate
    variations of exercises to keep
    your workouts fresh and
    challenge your muscles in new
    ways. For example, you can
    switch from barbell squats to
    goblet squats or from
    traditional push-ups to diamond
    push-ups.

5.3 Tracking Your Progress

Tracking your progress is vital to ensure that your workouts are effective and aligned with your goals.

Here are some key ways to track your progress:

1. **Keep a Workout Log**: Record the details of each workout, including exercises, sets, reps, and the amount of weight lifted. A workout log helps you track your progress over time and make informed adjustments to your routine.

2. **Measurements**: Take body measurements, such as waist circumference, hip circumference, and muscle size, to monitor changes in your physique.

3. **Body Weight**: Regularly weigh yourself under consistent conditions to track changes in body weight. Remember that weight can fluctuate daily due

to various factors, so focus on long-term trends.

4. **Performance Improvements**: Pay attention to how your strength and endurance improve over time. You should be able to lift heavier weights, perform more repetitions, or execute exercises with better form as you progress.

5. **Before and After Photos**: Take photos of your physique at the beginning of your fitness journey and at regular intervals. Visual progress can be motivating and provide insights into changes in your body composition.

6. **How You Feel**: Listen to your body. Note how you feel during and after workouts. Increased

energy levels, improved mood, and better sleep can be indicators of progress.

By tracking your progress, you can make data-driven decisions about your workout routine, allowing you to adjust and optimize your plan as you work toward your fitness goals.

creating a beginner-friendly workout routine involves careful planning, attention to progressive overload, and consistent tracking of your progress. With these principles in mind, you'll be well-equipped to embark on a successful weight training journey and achieve your fitness objectives.

CHAPTER 6

Proper Form and Technique

Maintaining proper form and technique during weight training exercises is of paramount importance for several reasons, including safety, effectiveness, and maximizing the benefits of your workouts.

6.1 Importance of Form

Proper form is critical for several reasons:

1. **Safety**: Ensuring you perform exercises with correct form reduces the risk of injury.

Weight training can be physically demanding, and improper technique can strain muscles and joints.

2. **Effectiveness**: Using proper form targets the intended muscle groups and helps you get the most out of each exercise. Correct technique ensures that the muscles you're trying to work are appropriately engaged.

3. **Progress**: Proper form promotes better progress. When you perform exercises incorrectly, you may not see the results you desire. It's through proper form that you can challenge your muscles effectively and stimulate growth.

4. **Long-Term Health**:
   Consistently using proper form
   helps maintain healthy joints,
   tendons, and ligaments. It also
   prevents overuse injuries that
   can occur when you repeatedly
   use improper technique.

5. **Efficiency**: Correct form
   allows you to lift heavier
   weights and perform more
   repetitions. This leads to
   increased strength and muscle
   development over time.

Quality always surpasses quantity in weight training. It's more important to perform an exercise with perfect form using a lighter weight than to lift a heavier weight with poor form.

6.2 Common Form Mistakes

Common form mistakes can compromise the safety and effectiveness of your weight training exercises. Recognizing and avoiding these errors is crucial. Some common form mistakes include:

1. **Using Momentum**: Swinging or using momentum to lift weights diminishes the engagement of the target muscles. It can also lead to injury. Maintain controlled movements throughout the exercise.

2. **Arching the Back**: Hyperextending your lower back during exercises like deadlifts and squats can lead to back injuries. Keep your back

straight and maintain a neutral spine.

3. **Round Shoulders**: Rounded shoulders during exercises like bench press can strain the shoulder joints. Keep your shoulders back and down.

4. **Improper Breathing**: Holding your breath during lifts can cause a spike in blood pressure. Breathe consistently, exhaling on the effort phase and inhaling on the return phase of the exercise.

5. **Overarching the Neck**: When doing overhead presses or similar exercises, avoid pushing your head forward. Keep your head in line with your spine.

6. **Overextending the Elbows**: Locking out your elbows

during exercises like bicep curls and tricep extensions can stress the joint. Maintain a slight bend in your elbows at the fully extended position.

7. **Rushing Through Repetitions**: Performing repetitions too quickly can compromise form and reduce the effectiveness of the exercise. Use controlled and deliberate movements.

8. **Neglecting Range of Motion**: Not completing the full range of motion can limit the benefits of the exercise. Ensure that you move through the entire range, even if it means using lighter weights.

6.3 How to Perform Exercises Correctly

To perform weight training exercises correctly and maintain proper form, follow these general guidelines:

1. **Start with a Stable Base**: Ensure your feet are shoulder-width apart or as needed for the exercise. A stable base provides balance and support.

2. **Engage Your Core**: Tighten your core muscles to stabilize your spine and protect your lower back.

3. **Maintain Neutral Spine**: Keep your spine in a neutral position, which means it should be straight without excessive arching or rounding.

4. **Controlled Movements**: Move
    the weight in a slow and
    controlled manner. Focus on
    the muscle you're targeting.

5. **Use a Full Range of Motion**:
    Move the weight through the
    complete range, allowing your
    muscles to fully contract and
    stretch.

6. **Proper Breathing**: Exhale
    during the effort phase of the
    exercise and inhale during the
    return phase.

7. **Use Proper Grip**: Grip the bar
    or dumbbells with a secure and
    comfortable grip to maintain
    control.

8. **Focus on the Mind-Muscle
    Connection**: Concentrate on
    the muscle group you're

working and feel it engaging throughout the exercise.

9. **Consult a Trainer**: If you're unsure about proper form, consider working with a qualified trainer who can provide guidance and feedback.

10. **Practice**: Practice makes perfect. Start with lighter weights to hone your form before progressing to heavier loads.

CHAPTER 7

Tips for Success

Achieving success in weight training involves more than just knowing the exercises and lifting weights. It also requires attention to essential aspects such as nutrition, recovery, and motivation.

7.1 Nutrition and Diet

Nutrition is a fundamental component of any successful weight training program. Your diet can significantly impact your progress, energy levels, and overall health. Here are some key nutrition tips:

1. **Balanced Diet**: Consume a balanced diet that includes a variety of foods from all food groups, including lean proteins, complex carbohydrates, healthy fats, fruits, and vegetables. This provides your body with essential nutrients for muscle growth and overall well-being.

2. **Protein Intake**: Ensure an adequate intake of protein to support muscle repair and growth. Lean sources of protein include chicken, turkey, fish, lean cuts of beef or pork, eggs, dairy, legumes, and plant-based protein sources like tofu and tempeh.

3. **Carbohydrates**: Carbohydrates provide energy for your workouts. Choose complex carbohydrates like whole

grains, oats, brown rice, and
sweet potatoes to sustain
energy levels during your
training sessions.

4. **Fats**: Healthy fats are crucial
   for overall health. Include
   sources of unsaturated fats,
   such as avocados, nuts, seeds,
   and olive oil, in your diet.

5. **Hydration**: Stay well-hydrated,
   as water is essential for muscle
   function and recovery.
   Dehydration can lead to
   decreased performance and
   muscle cramps.

6. **Meal Timing**: Eat balanced
   meals and snacks throughout
   the day to maintain steady
   energy levels. Consider having
   a meal with a mix of
   macronutrients about 1-2 hours

before your workout and a protein-rich meal or snack after your workout to support muscle recovery.

7. **Supplements**: While it's best to get nutrients from whole foods, some individuals may benefit from supplements like protein powders, creatine, or branched-chain amino acids (BCAAs). Consult with a healthcare professional or registered dietitian before using supplements.

8. **Caloric Intake**: If your goal is to build muscle, you may need to consume a surplus of calories to support growth. If your goal is weight loss, create a calorie deficit by monitoring your intake and increasing physical activity.

9. **Avoid Overeating**: While consuming sufficient nutrients is essential, avoid overeating, as excessive caloric intake can lead to weight gain. Portion control and mindful eating are key.

10. **Tracking and Adjusting**: Keep a food diary to monitor your eating habits and adjust your diet as needed to align with your goals.

7.2 Recovery and Rest

Proper recovery and adequate rest are just as important as your workouts. Here are tips for optimizing recovery:

1. **Sleep**: Aim for 7-9 hours of quality sleep per night. Sleep is

when your body repairs and grows muscle tissue.

2. **Active Recovery**: Engage in light physical activity on rest days. Activities like walking, swimming, or gentle yoga can aid recovery by increasing blood flow and reducing muscle soreness.

3. **Hydration**: Stay hydrated to support recovery processes. Water is crucial for flushing out waste products from your muscles.

4. **Nutrition**: After your workout, refuel with a balanced meal or snack that includes protein, carbohydrates, and healthy fats to aid muscle recovery.

5. **Stretching and Flexibility**: Incorporate stretching and

flexibility exercises into your routine to improve joint mobility and prevent muscle tightness.

6. **Foam Rolling and Self-Massage**: Use foam rollers or self-massage techniques to reduce muscle tension and promote circulation.

7. **Rest Days**: Incorporate regular rest days into your workout plan to allow your muscles time to recover and reduce the risk of overtraining.

8. **Stress Management**: High stress levels can hinder recovery. Practice stress management techniques like meditation, deep breathing, or mindfulness to support your well-being.

9. **Listen to Your Body**: Pay attention to signs of overtraining, such as persistent fatigue, decreased performance, and increased injury risk. Adjust your training intensity and volume as needed.

7.3 Staying Motivated

Maintaining motivation is often a challenge in any fitness journey. Here are some strategies to help you stay motivated:

1. **Set Realistic Goals**: Set achievable and specific goals that are aligned with your fitness aspirations. Having clear objectives can keep you focused.

2. **Progress Tracking**:
Continuously track your
progress, celebrate small
achievements, and use them as
motivation to keep going.

3. **Variety**: Change your workout
routine periodically to prevent
boredom and keep things fresh.
Try new exercises, classes, or
training methods.

4. **Find a Workout Buddy**:
Training with a friend or
workout partner can be
motivating and make your
workouts more enjoyable.

5. **Join a Fitness Community**:
Joining a fitness class or a
group that shares your interests
can provide accountability and
social support.

6. **Visualize Success**: Spend time
    visualizing your goals and the
    success you want to achieve.
    This can boost your motivation.

7. **Reward Yourself**: Consider
    setting up rewards for meeting
    your fitness milestones. These
    rewards can serve as positive
    reinforcement.

8. **Create a Schedule**: Establish a
    consistent workout schedule
    that becomes a part of your
    daily or weekly routine.

9. **Educate Yourself**: Learn about
    the benefits of exercise,
    nutrition, and how they impact
    your health. Knowledge can be
    motivating.

10. **Positive Self-Talk**: Replace
    negative self-talk with positive
    affirmations. Encourage

yourself and focus on your achievements.

11. **Music and Entertainment**: Create a workout playlist or listen to podcasts, audiobooks, or watch videos while exercising to make your workouts more enjoyable.

12. **Stay Consistent**: Understand that motivation can fluctuate, but consistency is key to long-term success. Push through days when motivation is low.

Focusing on nutrition, recovery, and motivation, you can enhance your success in weight training and maintain a fulfilling and sustainable fitness journey. These aspects complement your workouts and help you achieve your fitness goals effectively.

CHAPTER 8

Troubleshooting and Common Challenges

In your weight training journey, you may encounter various challenges that can hinder progress.

8.1 Dealing with Plateaus

Plateaus are common in weight training, and they occur when your progress seems to stall. Here's how to tackle plateaus:

1. **Change Your Routine**: One of the most effective ways to break through plateaus is to change your workout routine. Modify exercises, sets, reps, or

rest periods to provide your muscles with a new challenge.

2. **Increase Intensity**: Gradually increase the weight you lift. Progressive overload is essential for muscle growth, and lifting heavier weights can help you overcome plateaus.

3. **Vary Your Exercises**: Try different exercises that target the same muscle groups. This can stimulate muscle growth by working the muscles in a slightly different way.

4. **Focus on Form**: Ensure that your form is impeccable. Poor form can limit your progress, so pay close attention to technique.

5. **Rest and Recovery**: Ensure you're getting sufficient rest

and recovery. Overtraining can lead to plateaus, so incorporate rest days into your routine.

6. **Nutrition**: Reevaluate your diet to ensure you're getting the right nutrients to support muscle growth. Adjust your caloric intake if necessary.

7. **Mental Perspective**: A positive mindset can make a big difference. Believe in your ability to overcome plateaus and stay patient.

8. **Consult a Trainer**: If you're struggling with plateaus, consider consulting a qualified trainer who can help you adjust your workout plan and address specific challenges.

8.2 Avoiding Injuries

Injuries can be a setback in your weight training journey. Here's how to reduce the risk of injuries:

1. **Proper Form**: Always prioritize proper form and technique. Avoid using excessive weights that compromise your form.

2. **Warm-Up**: Always warm up before your workouts to prepare your muscles and joints for exercise.

3. **Cooldown and Stretching**: After your workout, engage in a cooldown and stretching routine to prevent muscle tightness.

4. **Strength Imbalances**: Address strength imbalances between

muscle groups to prevent overuse injuries. Incorporate exercises that target weaker areas.

5. **Listen to Your Body**: Pay attention to pain, discomfort, or unusual sensations. If something doesn't feel right, stop the exercise and seek guidance if needed.

6. **Rest and Recovery**: Ensure you're allowing enough time for rest and recovery to prevent overuse injuries and burnout.

7. **Progression**: Gradually increase the intensity and volume of your workouts to prevent sudden spikes in load that can lead to injuries.

8. **Footwear and Equipment**: Use appropriate footwear and

well-maintained equipment to prevent accidents or injuries.

9. **Cross-Training**: Incorporate cross-training activities to reduce the risk of overuse injuries. Engaging in different types of exercise can help balance muscle use and reduce strain.

8.3 Overcoming Mental Blocks

Mental blocks can impede your progress. Here are strategies to overcome mental barriers:

1. **Visualization**: Use visualization techniques to imagine yourself successfully completing challenging exercises. Visualization can

boost confidence and motivation.

2. **Goal Setting**: Set clear and achievable goals. Break down larger goals into smaller, more manageable milestones.

3. **Positive Self-Talk**: Replace negative self-talk with positive affirmations. Encourage yourself during challenging workouts.

4. **Mental Toughness**: Develop mental resilience and discipline. Understand that discomfort is part of the process, and your mental strength can carry you through it.

5. **Mindfulness and Meditation**: Practice mindfulness and

meditation to reduce anxiety and improve focus.

6. **Variety**: Change your routine periodically to prevent mental boredom. Trying new exercises or routines can keep your workouts interesting and mentally engaging.

7. **External Support**: Seek support from a workout buddy, a trainer, or a fitness community. The encouragement and accountability from others can help you stay motivated.

8. **Record Progress**: Keep a record of your progress to see how far you've come. This can be motivating and remind you of your accomplishments.

9. **Focus on the Present**: Don't dwell on past setbacks or worry about future obstacles. Focus on the present and the workout at hand.

10. **Remember Why**: Reflect on the reasons why you started your weight training journey in the first place. Reminding yourself of your motivations can reignite your commitment.

11. **Seek Professional Help**: If mental blocks persist and are affecting your progress, consider consulting a mental health professional or sports psychologist.

Addressing plateaus, avoiding injuries, and overcoming mental blocks, you can maintain a successful and fulfilling weight training journey.

These challenges are common, but with the right strategies and mindset, you can continue progressing toward your fitness goals.

8.4 Celebrating Your Achievements

Celebrating your achievements is a vital part of your weight training journey. Acknowledging your successes, no matter how small, can provide motivation, boost self-esteem, and keep you committed to your fitness goals. Here's how to effectively celebrate your achievements:

1. **Set Milestones**: Break your long-term fitness goals into smaller, achievable milestones. Each time you reach one of

these milestones, take a moment to celebrate.

2. **Record Your Progress**: Keep a detailed record of your workouts, including weights lifted, repetitions, and other metrics. Being able to see your progress in black and white can be incredibly motivating.

3. **Positive Reinforcement**: Use positive reinforcement as a celebration. For example, treat yourself to a healthy but delicious meal, a new workout outfit, or a massage after achieving a milestone.

4. **Visual Reminders**: Create visual reminders of your achievements. You can use progress photos, certificates, or

other visuals to remind yourself of your successes.

5. **Share with Others**: Sharing your achievements with friends, family, or your fitness community can be motivating and help you receive well-deserved recognition.

6. **Set New Goals**: As you achieve your milestones, set new, more challenging goals. The act of setting new targets can be a celebration of your progress.

7. **Reflect on Your Journey**: Take time to reflect on how far you've come in your fitness journey. Sometimes, we forget to appreciate our accomplishments when we're constantly striving for more.

8. **Internal Recognition**:
   Cultivate a sense of self-recognition. Acknowledge your hard work, dedication, and the improvements you've made, and take pride in your commitment to a healthier lifestyle.

9. **Consistency**: Celebrate the consistency of your efforts. Weight training and fitness are not just about grand achievements; they are also about consistently showing up and putting in the work.

10. **Motivation Boost**: Use the celebration of achievements as a motivation boost. It can remind you of your capacity for success and encourage you to keep pushing yourself.

celebrating your achievements is a personal and unique process. What matters most is that you take the time to appreciate your progress and acknowledge the effort you've put into your weight training journey. Celebrating achievements not only keeps you motivated but also reinforces your commitment to a healthier and stronger you.

www.ingramcontent.com/pod-product-compliance
Lightning Source LLC
Chambersburg PA
CBHW050835260726
48660CB00006B/2252